Battle Field Medical Force
– Planning For 21st Century Medical Readiness

Battle Field Medical Force – Planning For 21st Century Medical Readiness

Mohd Zin Bidin

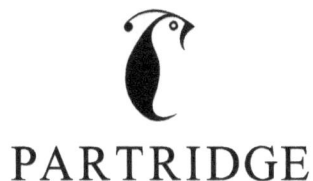

PARTRIDGE

Copyright © 2018 by Mohd Zin Bidin.

ISBN:	Softcover	978-1-4828-6560-8
	eBook	978-1-4828-6559-2

All rights reserved. No part of this book may be used or reproduced by any means, graphic, electronic, or mechanical, including photocopying, recording, taping or by any information storage retrieval system without the written permission of the author except in the case of brief quotations embodied in critical articles and reviews.

Because of the dynamic nature of the Internet, any web addresses or links contained in this book may have changed since publication and may no longer be valid. The views expressed in this work are solely those of the author and do not necessarily reflect the views of the publisher, and the publisher hereby disclaims any responsibility for them.

Print information available on the last page.

To order additional copies of this book, contact
Toll Free 800 101 2657 (Singapore)
Toll Free 1 800 81 7340 (Malaysia)
orders.singapore@partridgepublishing.com

www.partridgepublishing.com/singapore

Table of Contents

PREFACE		vii
PART 1	**INTRODUCTION**	1
Chapter 1	Introduction	3
PART 2	**MILITARY HEALTH CARE**	5
Chapter 2	Evolution of Military Health Services	7
Chapter 3	The Military Health Services System	9
	3.1 Echelons of Care	9
	3.2 Principles of Health Services Support	10
PART 3	**FIELD MEDICAL SERVICES**	13
Chapter 4	The Medical Battalion	15
Chapter 5	Planning for Medical Support in Operations	16
	5.1 Medical Planning Checklist	16
Chapter 6	Issues and Challenges Confronting Military Health Care	20
PART 4	**CONCEPT OF MEDICAL READINESS**	23
Chapter 7	Medical Readiness	25
	7.1 What does Readiness mean?	25
	7.2 Why do we need to measure Readiness?	26
	7.3 How does the Army measure Readiness?	27
Chapter 8	Medical Readiness in the Military Services	29
	8.1 What do Medics understand by the term Medical Readiness?	29
	8.2 Components of Medical Readiness	32

PART 5	FACTORS AFFECTING MEDICAL READINESS	35
Chapter 9	Medical Readiness – A Conceptual Framework	37
Chapter 10	Operational Aspect of Medical Readiness	41
	10.1 Inadequately Defined Missions	41
	10.2 Inadequate Training	42
Chapter 11	Administrative Aspect of Medical Readiness	45
	11.1 Lack of Top Management Commitment	45
	11.2 Out-dated Organisational Structure	47
	11.3 Shortage of Manpower	48
Chapter 12	Logistic Aspect of Medical Readiness	50
	12.1 Poor Logistics Support	50
	12.2 Poor Communication Networks	53

PART 6	ADDRESSING THE READINESS FACTORS	55
Chapter 13	Operational and Training Perspective	57
	13.1 Develop Well Defined Operational Mission	57
	13.2 Enhance Training	57
Chapter 14	Enhancing Management	61
	14.1 Change Management	61
	14.2 Balanced Scorecard	63
	14.3 Organisation Structure	64
	14.4 Improve Shortage of Personnel	65
Chapter 15	Improving Logistic and Communication	66
	15.1 Enhance Logistic Support	66
	15.2 Improve Communication Networks	67

PART 7	THE WAY FORWARD	69
Chapter 16	Planning for 21St Century Medical Readiness	71
Chapter 17	Conclusion	73

INDEX		79

PREFACE

Medical Readiness continues to be a persistent problem amongst militaries worldwide. It is essential that military services are well planned and have the capability to respond to the evolving changes of the battlefield environment. Planning for a Medical Support Operation is a complex procedure. Various factors need to be taken into account such as the complexity of warfare, rapid change in battlefield and mobility of medical resources as tactical situation changes. The provision of effective battlefield healthcare across the full spectrum of operational scenarios is an important requirement of today's Army. Military Health Care must be in the highest state of readiness, ready to be deployed within a short notice in any given situations.

This book attempts to crystallize the dynamics of Operation, Administration and Logistic and how they affect Medical Readiness. It highlights the challenges faced by frontline military medical units in the various areas of operations. It is organised according to major topics such as Military Health Care, Field Medical Services, Concepts of Medical Readiness and the Way Forward. Several management initiatives are proposed, and a Medical Readiness Concept Plan is developed. Key recommendations to enhance readiness are made.

Throughout the writing process, numerous articles, manuals and journals were used as references and several military medical experts were consulted. In-depth interviews were conducted with experienced individuals, focus groups and key informants, both from local and international. This book is written based on facts and suggestions, complemented with the author's extensive experience in Military Medicine. Due to the sensitivity of the subject, names of individuals, military units and countries have been kept anonymous.

I hope this book will be widely read by military leaders, doctors, medics and planners. I have written down facts based on extensive research and experiences of military medical practitioners worldwide.

Maj Gen Prof Dr Mohd Zin Bidin (Retd)
MD MPH MScCTM MScEBM FACTM(Hons)
FAOEMM FFTM FPHMM FFOM FAMM DTM&H psc

Founding Dean
Faculty of Medicine and Defence Health
National Defence University of Malaysia
December 2018

List of Figures

Figure 1: An Expanded Theoretical Framework of Medical Readiness — 38
Figure 2: Disaster and Military Medicine Simulation Centre – Proposed Building — 59
Figure 3: Training Facilities at the Disaster and Military Medicine Simulation Centre — 60
Figure 4: Floor Plan of the Disaster and Military Medicine Simulation Centre Comprising Jungle, Desert, Swamp and Disaster Environment — 60
Figure 5: Army Medicine Strategy Map — 63
Figure 6: A Proposed Organisational Structure for a Medical Battalion — 64
Figure 7: Seven Elements of Military Healthcare Supply Chain (Adopted from Basari, A.H.) — 67
Figure 8: Medical Readiness Concept Plan — 73

List of Tables

Table 1: Detailed Results for Factors Affecting Medical
　　　　　Readiness from the In-Depth Interviews　　　40
Table 2: Medical Readiness Problems and Recommendations　74

Abbreviations

ABBREVIATION	MEANING
ATLS	Advanced Trauma Life Support
BTLS	Basic Trauma Life Support
CIW	Counter Insurgency Warfare
EME	Electrical and Mechanical Engineer
GAQ	Operation, Administration, Logistic
HADR	Humanitarian Assistance and Disaster Relief
MINDEF	Ministry of Defence
OOTW	Operation Other than War
PESTLE	Political, Economic, Socio-Cultural, Technological, Legal and Environmental
SOAR	Strength, Opportunities, Aspiration, Result
SWOT	Strength, Weaknesses, Opportunity, Threat

PART 1
Introduction

CHAPTER 1
INTRODUCTION

"Leaders don't venture without vision. They don't pray without plan. They don't climb without clues. They are always prepared."

Israelmore Ayivor

    The changing face of warfare requires Medical Units to be deployed at a short notice, to the most hostile environment and with all its consequences. In whatever scenarios, medical care must be delivered to the troops to help the commander in the execution of his battle plan.

    The provision of good medical care is of immense value to the morale of the troops, knowing that they will be looked after if they are sick and wounded. Good medical care act as a combat multiplier, and can determine the consequences of war.

    Present day war scenarios require Medical units to be fast reacting, highly flexible and able to "deliver a greater medical capability of a higher quality" (Jenkin, 2004). The complexity of the battlefield environment and the speed of modern warfare will require an innovative, readily deployable and technologically sophisticated combat medical service. The services provided must be highly responsive and effective across the full spectrum of possible operational scenarios.

PART 2
Military Health Care

CHAPTER 2
EVOLUTION OF MILITARY HEALTH SERVICES

The history of Military Health Care dates back since countries started to wage war with each other. Medical services of British Army can be traced back to year 1660 when each regiment had its own Regimental Medical Officer (RMO) and his assistant (United Kingdom, Royal Army Medical Corps, u.d).

In the olden days, most victims of war died of diseases rather than injuries. The famous German commander, General Rommel, himself was evacuated twice from North Africa to Germany due to hepatitis. During this campaign, for every soldier who died of battle injury, three were lost due to diseases (Bellamy and Llewellyn, 1990). During the Soviet – Afghan War, 67% of the 620,000 Soviet troops had to be admitted to hospitals due to serious illnesses. It was also recorded that more than 3,000 men of the 5th Motorized Rifle Division was down with hepatitis (Grau and Jorgensen, 1997).

During the Cold War, most countries had large-scale combat medical services. However, with the increasing use of Rapid Deployment Forces, medical service will require innovative health support solutions. Today's scenarios demand smaller but more agile, flexible and highly mobile medical force, able to deliver greater medical capability of a higher quality (Jenkin, 2004).

Jenkin (2004) noted three key defence medical outputs which comprise trained and deployable medical capability, maintenance of fit personnel and the provision of prompt and effective healthcare. He suggested that today's military medical care should be able to treat a wide range of casualties and needs to be configured to respond to the demands of modern warfare. Military health care needs to prepare itself to respond promptly and professionally to provide the best healthcare to the fighting troops whenever and wherever they are deployed. Military health care units must be in the highest state of readiness at all times, ready to be deployed at a short notice to any place and at any time.

CHAPTER 3
THE MILITARY HEALTH SERVICES SYSTEM

The military health services are an important component of any military organisation. Its main objective is to conserve the fighting strength of the combat forces by providing operational health care in the battle areas. It supports the operational mission of the military by providing prevention, protection and treatment facilities across the whole spectrum of warfare.

3.1 Echelons of Care

In general, today's medical services of the Army consist of several levels or echelons of care. These are:

a. **Level 1** (First Responder) – Begin with the employment of first aid via self-aid or buddy aid. This is followed by paramedic emergency care, often under tactical environment in the forward edge of battle. Casualties are then evacuated to the Regimental Aid Post for further treatment by the Regimental Medical Officer.

b. **Level 2** (Forward Resuscitative Care) – This includes the capability to perform emergency medical treatment to save lives and limbs. This is normally provided by the forward hospital which is established by a company of the Medical Battalion).

c. **Level 3** (Field Hospital) – This is established by the Medical Battalion, and normally located at the Brigade

Maintenance Area. It has full theatre hospitalization capability.

d. **Level 4** (Armed Forces Hospital) – These consist of military and civilian general hospitals with full secondary and tertiary care facilities.

3.2 Principles of Health Services Support

The principles of health services support as proposed by USA Department of Army 2012 and adapted by several countries consist of:

a. Conformity – Medical support must be in conformity with the tactical plan.
b. Proximity – Medical assets must be placed within supporting distance of the supported manoeuvre forces, but not close enough to impede ongoing combat operations.
c. Flexibility – Medical resources must be prepared and empowered to shift medical resources to meet changing requirements or changes in tactical plan.
d. Mobility – Medical unit must be able to manoeuvre to ensure medical assets remain within supporting distance of the manoeuvring forces.
e. Continuity – Continuous care must be given throughout the chains of evacuation, extending from the point of injury to the support base.
f. Control – The Medical Commander must be in control of the medical assets to ensure scarce medical resources are efficiently employed to support the tactical and strategic plan.

It is apparent that providing a comprehensive combat medical care to support military operations is a complex task that requires concerted efforts and continuous planning. The medical support provided must be comprehensive and in consistence with the concept of operation. It must be highly flexible, mobile, agile and able to function in an austere environment, and ready to be deployed at a short notice.

PART 3
Field Medical Services

CHAPTER 4

THE MEDICAL BATTALION

In most countries, the provision of operational medical support is undertaken by the Medical Battalion. It is an Army unit under direct command of the Division Headquarters. The role of the Medical Battalion is to provide field medical support through:

a. Rapid clearance, evaluation and treatment of casualties.
b. Establishment of a mobile field or forward hospital with a bed capacity of 50 to 150.
c. Replenishment of essential medical supplies and equipment.
d. Augmenting the medical elements of the infantry battalion Regimental Aid Post (R.A.P).
e. Provision of preventive health services to enhance health and well being of the troops.

The Medical Battalion consist of specialised modules on wheels or in tentages, which can be deployed within a short time to areas of conflict. Each Battalion has three companies. Each medical company has a surgeon, an anaesthetist, five medical officers and about 50 paramedics. It has facilities in the form of operation theatre, X-Ray, laboratory, blood bank, induction & resuscitation room as well as dental and preventive medicine unit.

CHAPTER 5

PLANNING FOR MEDICAL SUPPORT IN OPERATIONS

Planning for a medical deployment is a complex procedure. It is essential to have a Medical Support Plan regardless of the type of military operations being supported (Bidin, 1993).

Medical Planner needs to consider the complexity of the operation, experience of the personnel, the likelihood of a rapidly changing battlefield and possibility of shifting Medical resources as the tactical situation changes (USA Department of Army, 1985).

In planning for a medical support operation, several factors have to be considered. The Australian Army Medical Corps (1983), United Kingdom Army Medical Corps (1950) and USA Department of Army (1985) and others have developed a format of checklist to consider when planning Medical Support Operations.

5.1 Medical Planning Checklist

a. Nature of Operation

Whether it is an assault, an advance, attack, defence or withdrawal, whether the fighting is to be open or close, whether the sea, land or air forces are engaged, these factors will dictate the number of wounded, and the medical facilities that need to be provided.

b. **Enemy Situation**

The Medical Commander must consider the enemy's ability to interfere with the Medical Support Operations such as his strength, disposition and combat efficiency.

c. **Friendly Situation**

It is important to determine the disposition of troops in order to decide the location of casualty densities and the best placement of supporting medical units.

d. **Characteristics of Areas of Operation**

Terrain. The type of terrain has the same bearing on Health Service Support planning as it does on tactical planning. Mountains, forests and swamps can be expected to constrain evacuation resources.
Climate. The Climate influences the incidence of diseases. It also determines measures for the prevention of disease, the scale and type of clothing required. Evacuation procedures, particularly by air are also highly influenced by weather conditions.
Flora and Fauna. Certain kinds of insects, animals and vegetation encountered in the area of operation may contribute to the non-effective rate of the command.

e. **Strength to be Supported**

The number of troops to be supported must be taken into consideration to estimate the size of health services support required.

f. Health of the Troops

This is an important consideration in making the Medical Support Plan. The Medical Commander needs to know the physical fitness of the troops, the level of morale, immunization status and status of training.

g. Casualty Estimate

Detailed estimate must be done with regard to number, distribution, areas of patient density, and lines of evacuation. This will enable the requirements for medical support in terms of location, numbers and types of treatment to be planned.

h. Time and Space

Medical capabilities must take into account time and space considerations. These include evacuation distances, speed and turnaround time of evacuation vehicles, and time needed for collection and treatment of casualties.

i. Resources Available

Having determined the above factors, the Medical Commander then considers the resources on hand or readily available to meet the requirements. Following a comparison between the requirements and the resources actually available, a decision is made as to the sufficiency (or otherwise) of the available resources to accomplish the aim. If not, additional resources are requested. If no additional resources are available, and operations have to go on, infantry commander must be told that troop's safety will be compromised.

In an effort to enhance Medical Readiness, the military medical service must consider the above planning factors when designing its support plan. However, the changing nature of war will make medical planning difficult. Salisbury and English (2003) noted that modern warfare will not only change the number and nature of casualties, but also change their distribution on the battlefield. Traditional methods of distributing battlefield healthcare support will no longer be efficient and effective.

CHAPTER 6

ISSUES AND CHALLENGES CONFRONTING MILITARY HEALTH CARE

There have been persistent Medical Readiness problems amongst militaries worldwide. Even the US Army medical units face several problems such as not being prepared for the assigned war missions, outdated mobilization plan, undeployable medical personnel and insufficient logistic support (USA General Accounting Office, 1995). These problems called for radical changes to reform the system in the face of the 21st Century.

Joseph (1995) proposed several management initiatives to reform military healthcare in order to support the various spectrums of military operations. The objectives include, among others, to:

a. Ensure the medical structure has a robust, seamless and assured communication capability within the global communication architecture.
b. Develop a modern medical information system.
c. Keep medical logistics organizations at pace with new defence strategies and logistic demands.
d. Develop and update acquisition and support plans that support the full spectrum of military operations.
e. Provide comprehensive medical logistic information management and communication systems.
f. Ensure timely availability of required personnel or units to accomplish the medical evacuation mission.

g. Develop and execute programs to procure and/or modernize evacuation platforms.
h. Recruit and retain qualified active and reserve personnel to meet military medical requirement by specialty and grade.
i. Mobilize reserve component medical forces to integrate with active duty forces.
j. Establish common medical training guidelines, policies, and standards to promote medical readiness.
k. Utilize field medical training sites to enhance interoperability and shared training.

In preparing for 21st century Medical Readiness, the Army must take into considerations the above proposals and try to adapt some of the initiatives. Factors identified in this study that hinder Medical Readiness must be addressed at the strategic and operational level.

The complexity of battlefield healthcare and the changing nature of war demands a thorough planning and concerted effort by all relevant stakeholders. Over the years, military organisations have questioned the capacity and capability of military health units in providing quality health care in the combat operations. Several issues were raised such as inexperienced staff, out of date equipment, slow in reacting and inappropriate support for specific operations.

Elsewhere, the US General Accounting Office (1995) reported about problems with deployed medical units which were neither adequately staffed nor equipped to fulfil the wartime missions. The report expressed its concern about Department of Defence's ability to meet its wartime mission and described problems such as inadequate training, missing equipment and the large number of non-deployable personnel as serious threats to the Department's ability to provide adequate medical support to deployed forces. It also highlighted several readiness issues such as inability of medical unit to provide medical care to support the evacuation of casualties and to treat large numbers of chemically contaminated casualties. Other issues highlighted include misassignment of personnel, insufficient training, incompatible communication equipment, shortfalls in transportation assets and poor management of war reserves. The report summarises factors affecting Medical Readiness which can be attributed to:

a. Out of date, untested, and invalidated mobilization plan.
b. Undeployable medical personnel due to poor physical conditions, insufficient training, lack of required skills and mismatch in medical specialties.
c. Insufficient or missing medical equipment and supplies

The three factors above can be examined from operational, administrative and logistics perspective, as proposed in the theoretical framework.

PART 4
Concept of Medical Readiness

CHAPTER 7

MEDICAL READINESS

7.1 What does Readiness mean?

According to the American Heritage Dictionary (2000), readiness is the state of being fully "prepared or available for service or action". It implies availability for immediate use or action.

The Random House Kernerman Webster's College Dictionary (2010) defines readiness as "the condition of being ready; ready for action or movement; promptness, quickness, willingness."

The Picturesque Thematic Dictionary describes readiness as "all systems go, all set, everything's ready, let us roll". It also means "availability, willingness, readiness, eagerness, desirousness, to be prepared for any possibility, to be armed and ready to fight, raring to go". The Dictionary of Military and Associated Terms defines readiness as "the ability of the military force to fight and meet the demands of the national military strategy, whereas unit readiness is the ability to provide capabilities required by the combatant commanders to execute their assigned missions." Joint readiness is further defined as the "combatant commander's ability to integrate and synchronize ready combat and support forces to execute his or her assigned missions."

In the military medical context, most of the definitions can be applied provided the word "fighting" is omitted. As a unit, the Medical Battalion must always be prepared and available for service. It must always be ready for action with promptness, quickness and willingness. It must be prepared for any possibility, raring to go, to meet the demands of the national military strategy. It must be immediately available.

7.2   Why do we need to measure Readiness?

The Army measures readiness to verify whether it is ready to go to war and to see how effectively it can conduct the war. It aims to check whether the unit's preparation in terms of personnel, training and logistics are adequate.

The Medical Battalion, being an army unit itself needs to assess its capability and make a decision with regards to its deployability and employability.

According to Peltz et al (2002), the Army measures readiness to:

a. Assess the readiness of Army Equipment in the event it is needed for an actual deployment, is the equipment ready to go?
b. Understand how well the Army could sustain equipment in different situations in which its use is anticipated. When the equipment is deployed and then employed, how well can the Army keep it working?
c. Detect changes in logistics support performance and failure rates. Are any problems developing Army-wide?
d. Understand what drives the Army capabilities to keep equipment operational and where there are long term problems in sustaining equipment.

Similarly, the Medical Battalion needs to measure readiness to ensure its assets are ready for deployment, and when deployed, they must be kept operational. Medical Battalion needs to ensure it has the right mix of personnel, the correct equipment and the appropriate strategy to perform its combat support function. For this to happen, it needs to review its vision and mission. The Medical Battalion needs to review its structure, equipment and doctrine, to bring about transformational change in order to enhance its readiness capability. These changes need to align with the present political, economical, social, technological, legal, and environmental scenarios.

According to Junor (2005), military planners are now shifting the focus from reporting unit readiness to managing joint force capabilities. This will imply a shift from resources to capabilities where combined forces, are all contributing to front- line operations. Forces are not just supposed to be ready but must be able to adapt to meet the current needs of warfare.

7.3 How does the Army measure Readiness?

As a member of the Army force, the Medical Battalion is required to measure readiness in accordance to the Army formula. Readiness in the Army is measured as the percentage of a given assets that is fully functional. It must be noted that capability is not synonymous with readiness. A highly capable force is not necessarily be ready for deployment.

In the Malaysian Army according to Nor (2003), "readiness is measured based on the elements of strength of the personnel, communication, mobility, logistics, training and firepower, whereas capability is the available strength over actual strength. These definitions are shown in the formula below:

$$\text{Readiness} = \frac{\text{Equipment fully mission capable}}{\text{Actual strength}} \quad \frac{\text{(Serviceability)}}{\text{(Actual Strength)}}$$

$$\text{Capability} = \frac{\text{Available strength}}{\text{Actual strength}} \quad \frac{\text{(Holding)}}{\text{(Actual Strength)}}$$

The above measurements, while easy to understand, assume that all elements in the category contribute the same amount to readiness. It does not take into account other intangible factors such as nature of operations, morale, tactic, leadership style, terrain, climate, and the various war scenarios under which the unit is deployed.

It should be further noted that the measurement techniques used here are the legacy of Army information systems which were developed during the old days of computer technology when computers have limited memory, speed was slow and capability limited. (Peltz, Robin et al, 2002). With the development of information technology, measurement of readiness will become more comprehensive and complicated.

Peltz, et al (2002), propose that Army must have comprehensive metrics that measure equipment readiness capabilities that portrays the interaction between equipment reliability to equipment readiness.

The central issues discussed above focus on the aspect of operations, administrative and logistics and how they affect readiness. Various aspects have been discussed, formulas advocated and methodology developed. Up to this date, there is no perfect way to measure readiness.

CHAPTER 8

MEDICAL READINESS IN THE MILITARY SERVICES

8.1 What do Medics understand by the term Medical Readiness?

Medical Readiness means different things to different people. This in-depth interview with several senior military Medical doctors and enlisted men has enabled the concept of Medical Readiness to be delved further.

A, B and C denote interviewees recorded for the study. Their identities and countries of origin have been kept confidential.

One interviewee suggested that Medical Readiness is the *"state of functional and operational capability of a unit to perform its assigned mission"*. *(A2)* Another spoke of the *"ability of a group of trained and competent individuals, given the right equipment and method, to respond to a situation within the appropriate time frame"*. *(C1)* Others mentioned about the *"ability of a unit to execute its main mission given the right manpower, materials and methods."* Several interviewees mentioned about the *"need to have continuous, efficient and reliable supply chain, standardized and well-maintained equipment, standardized operating procedures and the right men for the right job."* *(A1, A6, A9, B1, C2)*

The above concept is in consonant with several definitions and concepts described in several military literatures. This concept is different from *individual medical readiness* which comprises periodic medical examination, laboratory studies and limiting conditions for deployment of individual soldiers (USA Air Force Instruction, 2007).

Whilst individual health status is important for overall unit readiness, the fact, remains that overall battlefield healthcare has often been neglected, and remains a fundamental problem in many Armies of the world. It is against this backdrop that this study is devoted to.

The central issue addressed here is the readiness of the Medical Battalion to render its operational health services to the deployed troops. This can be in the war zones, in areas of conflict or in places of disaster. A ready Medical Force will ensure that every deployed soldiers will be taken care of if they are injured. Such medical unit will be capable of performing its assigned task, whether in battles, or in Humanitarian and Disaster Response Operations (HADR). This is what most respondents understand about readiness of the Medical Battalion.

Most respondents do not know how the figures were obtained. However, they were quick to give their reasons for the low state of readiness. All respondents mentioned about shortage of manpower and poor logistics support. *"When these are in shortages, readiness will surely go down"*, they said. *(A1, A2, A6, A9, B1, C2)*

State of readiness of a unit is a sensitive matter. A figure does not mean much unless we know what are the parameters measured and how they interphase with each other. Furthermore, a figure may not indicate capability of equipment to support the army vision (Peltz et al 2002). The question is not just what forces are capable of, but how well they can meet current operational needs (Junor, 2005).

It is evident that Medical Readiness is affected by several quantitative and qualitative factors. Whilst it is easy to measure the strength or stocks of personnel and equipment, it is more complex to measure morale, skills, relationships, quality of care and best practices. Bearing this in mind, this book attempts to explore the above factors in a more systematic manner. The factors identified from the literatures and in-depth interviews help to explain the complexity of Medical readiness in an operational environment. These factors include, among others, leadership, morale of personnel, capability of enemy, skill of healthcare providers, availability of supplies, unit manning level, lines of communication, mobilization capability and personal and family issues. For discussion purposes, these factors are grouped under operation, administration and logistics.

Within the above complex, clandestine and diverse setting of the military environment, it is not surprising why the subject of Medical Readiness is not much discussed in the literature. Every military medical community does some measurements, but no one shares their results. There is not even a clear definition to describe readiness from the medical viewpoint. It is assumed that everyone understands the term. The few articles written on Medical Readiness focus only on *Individual Medical Readiness* rather total medical force readiness.

Individual readiness is concerned about the health condition, fitness level, immunisation status and psychological profile of individual soldiers. Individual Medical Readiness is not Medical Force Readiness. It is only one of its components. Medical Readiness in military setting is the capability of the military medical unit to be deployed for a specified operation, at a specified duration, to perform the assigned task for which it is organised to do. This task must commensurate with its structure. A Medical Battalion established to support troops for a Counter Insurgency warfare cannot be expected to operate in a large conventional environment.

It is accepted that the Medical Battalion is also responsible for ensuring health of the troops (force health protection) and implement preventive public health measures in the battlefield. In other words, it is expected to perform preventive and curative tasks. This will even make the measurements of readiness more complex and demanding.

8.2 Components of Medical Readiness

Kasper and Klein (2000) proposed several key monitoring and surveillance functions which may provide important measures of Medical Readiness. These measures include:

a. Assessment of overall health readiness status of troops through medical situation reports.
b. Establishment of an epidemiological surveillance data – collection and reporting system.
c. Verification of a system for the management of stress and prevention of post-traumatic stress disorder.
d. Certification of the readiness of friendly nations' deployed medical capabilities.
e. Assessment of the medical force protection function which will provide commanders with an assessment of the readiness of the medical support structure at all levels.
f. Provision of selected force protection preventive medical training.

To put it in another way, apart from the provision of emergency medical care, measurement of Medical Readiness should take into considerations preventive and public health measures, medical training, psychological preparation and support from military medical teams of friendly nations.

Kasper and Klein (2000) also proposed the inclusion of preventive medical measures as part of operational plans. These measures among others include the:

a. Identification of risk for terrain, climate, endemic diseases, special environmental and occupational hazards.

b. Identification of preventive and controlling measures, including policy on immunization and prophylactic measures.
c. Advising and auditing the quality of waters and food.

The above measures are essential for Medical Readiness and must be included in the operational planning process. They must be implemented throughout the pre-deployment, deployment, and post-deployment phase. It is the responsibility of the Medical Battalion to comply with the preventive medicine measures. Medical staff of the Battalion must advice commanders and troops on the importance of field and personnel health as this will contribute to the overall Medical Readiness of the Unit.

PART 5

Factors Affecting Medical Readiness

CHAPTER 9

MEDICAL READINESS – A CONCEPTUAL FRAMEWORK

Various factors must be identified when discussing about medical readiness. These include mobilizations plans, enemy situations, characteristics of areas of operations, casualty estimate, enemy tactics, time and space etc. These can be grouped under the categories of Operation (G factor), Administration (A factor) and Logistics (Q factor). G factor includes strategies and tactics of warfare. Administration (A factor) includes things such as manpower, leadership, management, skill of personnel, morale, motivation and others. The Logistics (Q factor) include transport, supply, communication sets, tentages, furniture, drugs, medical equipment and the long list of healthcare supply chain.

The book attempts to crystallize the dynamics of Operation, Administration and Logistics and how they affect Medical Readiness. As a consequence of this, a theoretical framework is proposed as shown in Figure 1.

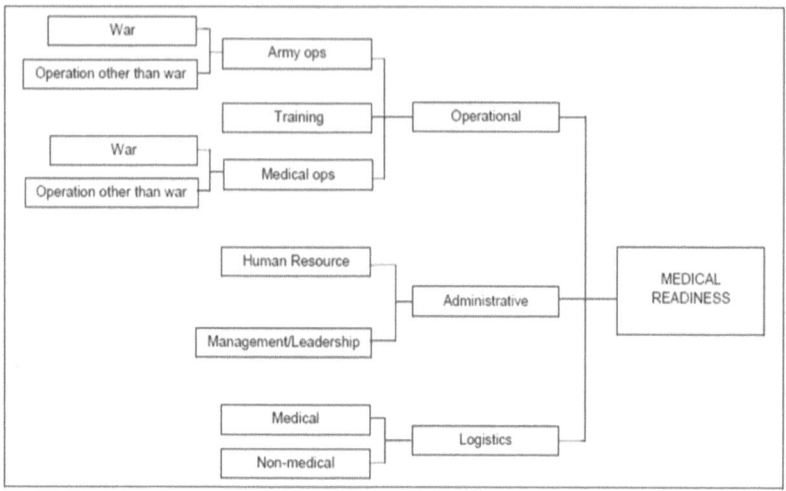

Figure 1: An Expanded Theoretical Framework of Medical Readiness

In general, factors affecting Medical Readiness can be classified as follows:

Operational Factors

- Type and nature of operations.
- Inadequately defined mission.
- Lack of strategic planning.
- Inappropriate deployment for non-core functions.

Administrative Factors

- Misassignment of personnel.
- Undeployable personnel.
- Poor manning level.
- Lack of knowledge and skill.
- Lack of standard operating procedures.
- Out-dated organisational structure.
- Inadequate training.

Logistics Factors

- Shortfalls in equipment.
- Poor maintenance and serviceability.
- Poor supply chain.
- Obsolescent equipment.
- Poor communication networks.

This book focused on the following critical factors namely:

a. Inadequately Defined Missions.
b. Inadequate Training.
c. Lack of Top Management Commitment.
d. Out-dated Organisational Structure.
e. Shortage of Manpower.

f. Poor Logistics Support.
g. Poor Communication Networks.

These factors are selected based on in depth interviews with experienced individuals, focus groups and key informants with extensive operational experiences.

	INTERVIEW SUB ISSUES	A1	A2	A3	A4	A5	A6	A7	A8	A9	A10	B1	B2	B3	B4	B5	B6	C1	C2
G FACTORS	INADEQUATELY DEFINED MISSION	√	√	•	•	*	√	√	√	*	√	√	*	*	√	√	√	√	*
	INADEQUATE TRAINING	*	*	*	*	*	*	√	√	*	*	√	√	√	√	√	√	*	*
A FACTORS	LACK OF TOP MANAGEMENT COMMITMENT	*	*	*	*	*	√	√	*	*	√	*	*	*	√	√	√	*	*
	OUT-DATED ORGANISATIONAL STRUCTURE	*	*	*	√	√	*	√	√	*	•	√	√	√	√	•	•	√	√
	SHORTAGE OF MANPOWER	*	*	√	•	√	√	*	*	√	√	*	*	*	√	•	*	√	*
Q FACTORS	POOR LOGISTICS SUPPORT	*	*	*	√	√	*	√	*	*	*	*	*	*	*	√	√	*	*
	POOR COMUNICATION NETWORKS	*	*	√	√	√	√	*	*	•	√	√	√	√	√	√	√	•	•

Key:
    A, B, C are interviewees
    *   Interviewee confirmed as relevant
    √   Interviewee implied as relevant
    •   Not mentioned

Table 1: Detailed Results for Factors Affecting Medical Readiness from the In-Depth Interviews

CHAPTER 10

OPERATIONAL ASPECT OF MEDICAL READINESS

10.1 Inadequately Defined Missions

The main objective of the Medical Battalion is to conserve the fighting strength of the combat forces. Over the years of its existence, the battalion has been engaged into various roles it never expected to perform. To illustrate, besides its primary role, the Battalion has been deployed to provide humanitarian assistance for the numerous disasters that have occurred in the region. The battalion was also involved in Medical standby for the major sports events such as the Commonwealth Games, Asian Games and even the World Motorsports events such as the Formula 1 and Motorcycle Grandprix. While these have enhanced the reputation of the Army in general, the Medical Battalion is left with this inherent pressure of an open-ended expansion of Medical mission.

The lack of strategic guidance that clearly defines the requirements and rules of engagement of these missions may lead to confusion, ambiguity and a state of unpreparedness. It would be fitting and proper if top commanders first consider which missions are appropriate for military medical deployment, make assessment and decide whether it is adequately prepared for it. It is worth noting that medical support requirements for these events differ from combat operation. Furthermore, the old structure of the battalion does not permit it to have a robust and flexible system that can meet a broad range of Medical demands.

Whilst those secondary medical support operations may put a lot of pressures on the Battalion's personnel and assets, most respondents have no objections in taking part. Some mentioned about monetary gains, promotions, medals and recognition by peers as reasons for participating. Others mentioned about the experience and the preparation that mimics a war deployment. *"This type of operation mimics a true deployment in wartime situation" (A7)*, says a senior officer who has been deployed to several non-combat missions. *"Personnel have the experience of treating injured patients in the field, working with limited resources in an austere environment" (A5)*. Whatever the rationale behind these missions, the core business of the battalion must not be compromised. The staff should not be deployed just for deployment sake. Proper equipment must be made available and personnel must be adequately trained. Perhaps it would be ideal if the battalion has a specialised team, equipped with modular, deployable and special purpose packages for these specific missions. In this way, readiness for core military functions would not be compromised.

10.2 Inadequate Training

Training is a form of instruction, discipline or drill, to be taught so as to make fit, qualified, or proficient, or to be made prepared (as by exercise / learning) for a test or skill, towards an aim or an objective set by the organisation (Basari H, 2009).

It is the acquisition of knowledge, through learning specific skills to enhance one's capability and performance. The Collins English Dictionary defines training as "the process of bringing a person to an agreed standard of proficiency, by practice and instruction."

In the military environment, training is divided into individual and collective training. Medical personnel have to undergo both military and medical specialty training. In spite of the importance of training, the fact remains that the Medical Battalion does not meet its training requirements to sustain and enhance its readiness. These are due to factors such as shortage of manpower, lack of instructors, frequent deployments, lack of facilities, and lack of relevant curriculum.

> *"Training is inadequate. It needs improvement,"* said a respondent. *(C1)*

> *"Our personnel are not competent in clinical skills. We need to send them to the nearby government hospital for training". (A9)*

> *"We are medics. We don't know war tactics". (A9)*

> *"Our diploma holders do not know basic nursing skills. They are not clever. They have attitude and discipline problem. They have no interest to learn". (A9)*

> *"Our doctors should attend courses in Advanced Trauma Life Support, Basic Cardiac Life Support, Advanced Cardiac Life Support, Pre-hospital Care and Combat Casualty Care". (A9)*

Those are worthwhile information on the gaps of knowledge that exist among the medical personnel. In fact this gap exists amongst all members of the Medical Corps.

Training in the battalion must be enhanced and given top priority. New courses and relevant curriculum must be developed to cater for the gaps in knowledge and skill of members of the battalion. Lists of relevant courses such as ATLS, BTLS and Combat Casualty Care must be conducted. Professional enhancement programs to enhance the clinical skills of unit personnel must be implemented. As for military related training, the Army must be consulted to design relevant programs to enhance military healthcare skill in combat operations.

Whilst most respondents emphasised the importance of training, there seem to be little effort on the part of the Battalion to enhance it. Several programs have been proposed by the Commanding Officer, but approval from top management is still pending.

CHAPTER 11

ADMINISTRATIVE ASPECT OF MEDICAL READINESS

11.1 Lack of Top Management Commitment

Of all the factors that affect Medical Readiness, *top level commitment* ranks highest in the list. Almost all respondents gave prominence to this element as the most critical factor that will give the greatest impact on unit preparedness. Without top level commitment, it is going to be very difficult to implement any process that can have any significant change in the Battalion. This is especially so in the Military culture where the *General decides on everything.*

Military doctors of the Army, mostly holding mid-level position in the Divisional Command are in agreement on this issue. They feel that they are being abandoned and neglected, and there is nothing they can do about it. *"Without top level commitment, we will always be stucked in this situation, always not ready, operating with minimal structure, inadequate assets and unclear direction. I am afraid the Army just washes their hands on this matter and leave it to the Medical Corps to handle"*, said an interviewee. *(A1)*

Being an Army Unit under the Divisional Command, the Medical Battalion in most countries reports to the Brigade Headquarters for operational, administrative and logistics matters. The Medical Headquarters only has technical command over the Battalion, advising on matters of healthcare and personnel. Procurement, maintenance and repair of major equipment such as vehicles, ambulances, telecommunications sets, furniture, tentages etc are under the purview of the Army Command. Maintenance and Maintenance Support Plan is the Army's responsibility. Within these diverse and complex setting, the Medical Battalion is always *at a lost* compared to the Infantry Unit. The battalion is always given last priority. This is expected, as the core business of the Army is to fight the enemy and they must be provided with superior firepower. More allocation is given to purchase weapons rather than medical equipment. Furthermore, all Division Commanders are themselves former infantry officers, who may be biased towards their own corps.

As for the military doctors, understanding the uniqueness of the military culture is something they learned late in their professional carrier. Developing rapport with the top management is something intricate and complex for them. Moreover, commander's preferred style of command is sometimes alien or unfamiliar to the medical fraternity. This leads to a distant relationship between Commanders and Doctors, resulting in a cold, rigid and uncordial relationship. If this situation persists, support from major stakeholders such as the Ordnance, Engineer and Service Corps will be difficult to come by. In this context, it would be useful to remind Military Commanders on the important role they play to ensure the Medical Battalion is capable to support his troop in battle. The Army Commanders at a higher level of command should *"appreciate the services given by the Medical Battalions and should give similar priority as that given to an infantry battalion"*, says one respondent. *(C2)*

Perhaps, a deeper understanding of the process of Medical Service Support by the commander and a good understanding of the art of warfare by military doctors will go a long way in enhancing commander – doctor relationship. The Army needs to make Medical Readiness as one of the Commander's Key Performance Indicator (KPI). This will help in a long way to obtain continuous top level commitment. Otherwise, medical service will always remain *notional*, where its presence is just imaginary and wishful thinking.

11.2 Out-dated Organisational Structure

The Medical Battalion of most countries inherits its structure from the old *Field Surgical and Transfusion Team* (FSTT), a World War 2 medical establishment. The emerging threat of conventional warfare with weapons of mass destruction require a comprehensive review of the Medical Battalion.

With the end of the Cold War, the Armed Forces of several countries embarked on modernising its conventional warfare capability. However, the Medical Battalion remained as it was, to cater for CIW. To make matters worse, the Medical Battalion is required to be multitasking, multiskilling and need to be on standby to perform tasks it may not be capable of doing.

It is important to highlight that an organisation of such a structure cannot be expected work wonders in an era of modern technology and a world of uncertainties. Organisational structure, according to Llyod (undated), is much like a human skeleton. It determines what shape an organisation will take, and it can be the underlying cause of a problem.

Being a military organisation, the Medical Battalion has too many levels of hierarchy which become barriers to empowerment. Decisions have to pass through several levels of command before any decisions are made. One respondent trying to get an ambulance repaired was quoted as saying *"We have to go to the EME workshop, then to Ordnance, then to Service Corps. As customers, we want a one- stop shopping centre. One person to get all our needs done. Here, request takes months or years". (A1)* It seems that the team members of the unit were complaining about all sorts of problems – poor maintenance, poor communication, limited manpower, and lack of skills and a host of other problems.

A closer look at the root causes will disclose that the *structure is actually the problem.* How can a Medical Battalion, originally established to support a Division in a low intensity conflict, end up looking after Divisions engaged in Conventional, Counter-Insurgency and Humanitarian Assistance and Disaster Relief Operations?

So it is wise to look back at the organisation structure. It might be the main problem no one thought about. It might be worth investing time and money, redesigning an effective and efficient structure for the Medical Battalion. This can be structured in different ways, such as by:

   a. Functions – e.g. Casualty evacuation, resuscitation, surgery, radiology etc.
   b. Region or division – e.g. 1 battalion for each division, 1 medical company for each Brigade.
   c. Work teams – e.g. Forward Surgical Team, Preventive Medicine Team, Medical Intelligence Team, Sports Medicine Team, HADR Team, Rapid Deployment Team etc.

It is worth suggesting that the Battalion should be less hierarchical and more flat, with just one person in charge with other key personnel reporting to him on an equal levels. This is common in the medical professions where each specialist wants to be his own boss in his department. This will create better communication, better team spirit and faster decision making. *"Structure of the organisation needs to be revised to adequately cover the operational requirements of the Armed Forces". (A6)*

11.3 Shortage of Manpower

In order to be able to provide optimum care for the combat forces, the Medical Battalion must be adequately manned. Often times, there are shortage of deployable medical personnel, and this can lead to reduced capability to render battlefield healthcare.

Shortages of personnel can prevent optimal use of available healthcare facilities and resources. Even if all vacancies are filled, shortages will still occur as wartime requirements may be caught short of the right mix of qualified and experienced personnel. Most of medical personnel are unique to the military and have no equivalence in their civilian counterpart. Even the medics who render first line medical care at the battle fronts are exclusive individuals, unparalleled in the civilian medical profession. This being the case, it is important for the Army to have a wartime staffing plan to solve this perennial problem.

Shortages of medical personnel are greatest in the various specialties such as surgery, anaesthesiology, orthopaedic, radiology and traumatology. Even among the nurses, shortages occur in areas such as intensive care, surgery and emergency care. Other allied health personnel such as optometrist, audiologist, physiotherapist and psychologist are not part of the Battalion organisation, even though their services are of operational importance.

For years the Army field operational service has encountered these manpower problems, and there has been no significant effort to solve it. In fact the problem has got worse due to budget cut in most countries. This shortage is further compounded when Medical Battalion personnel are required to be attached to the Military Hospitals while some have to provide medical covers even for unimportant events. *"Just in November this month, the Battalion has been tasked to provide medical standby for a youth motivational camp, dinner night and Army sports events. These are of no benefit, irrelevant and a waste in terms of time and money,"* said an interviewee *(B2)*. Another respondent added, *"the time could have been used to conduct collective training to enhance the Battalion's readiness." (A3)*

CHAPTER 12

LOGISTIC ASPECT OF MEDICAL READINESS

12.1 Poor Logistics Support

Logistics requirement for the Medical Battalion can be divided into Operational Logistics and Medical Logistics. Operational Logistics comprise transport, generators, furniture, spares, and food services. These are normally provided by specialised logistics corps such as the Ordnance Corps, Services Corps, the Electric and Mechanical Engineer Corps (EME), the Signal Corps and the Engineer Corps. These are all Army Corps, each with their own inherent problems. As long as the Medical Battalion relies on them for field logistics support, readiness will not improve. This is evident from the interviews where almost all respondents agreed that they did not get adequate supply from the field logistic services. Some of the respondents' comments are as follows:

> "Army logistics procedure is not suitable for us. Obsolete Equipment and vehicles, lack of maintenance, lack of priority for Medical Battalion are perennial problems". (A1)

> "These poor logistics supports had reduced the battalion's capabilities". (A9)

> "These problems create a lot of uneasiness, inappropriate anxiety and stress to us. We can't do anything with the Army Log". (A9)

> "It is glaring clear that we don't have the adequate number of ambulances to support the Casualty Evacuation Units. The ones that we have are very old and often break down. They lack speed and do not have off-road capabilities". (A1)

> "The Army must be committed to develop and maintain our assets and supplies". (C2)

> "The present logistics doctrine does not work and needs to be modified". (A9)

> "To deploy a Medical Company alone, we need 30 x 3 ton trucks. Without enough vehicles, how can we have readiness?" (B3)

> "Armies that neglect logistics will lose the wars". (A3)

> "Deployment time has always been delayed because of logistics". (A8)

The quotes come from men on the ground, and can go on and on, but suffice to say, logistics really has a great impact on readiness. It is of great importance that basic vehicles and equipment must be provided before capability can be enhanced.

On the other hand, Medical Logistics is under the purview of the Medical Headquarters in Mindef. The provision of this support requires collaboration between the clinicians and the medical logistician. Medical logistics encompasses medical materiel, medical equipment maintenance and repair, medical gases, blood storage and distribution, and medical contracting support.

Medical Logistics is different from line logistics. Medical products and services used by the military medical services are critical to the success of medical missions (USA Department of Army, 2009). Individuals looking after this function must be able to anticipate what the user needs based on the peculiarities of the operations. Non availability of certain equipment can be detrimental.

The extensiveness of these specific commodities is reflected in the list of items such as flammable and corrosive items, controlled medical items, fragile items requiring special storage, handling and packaging, and medical gases (USA Department of Army, 2000).

Medical unit must be provided with the latest medical capability to attain a high standard of care expected by the combat troops. This will tell the troops that the nation cares about them. At the present time, the capability of Medical Logistics to support troops in the full spectrum of operation needs to be looked into. Several comments by the interviewees will attest to this:

> "We need to gather medical items from the hospitals to establish the Battalion field hospital". (B3)

> "We have no prepacked medical drugs and equipment available for rapid deployment". (A6)

> "There is no standardised Medical equipment allocated to each battalion". (A6)

> "The equipment is not well maintained and never calibrated". (B3)

"To my knowledge, there has never been any military exercise where the healthcare supply chain has been tested". (A6)

"We need time to load medical assets. Stocks are limited. Sometimes the same equipment is being used for all sorts of medical covers". (B1)

"We only got half of what we requested". (B4)

"The Medical Battalion has no biomedical engineering services". (B6)

"Many departments in the forward hospital are not fully equipped". (B4)

"The top management only gives priority to hospital services. Field medical services have long been neglected". (A9)

These are logistics issues pertinent to the Medical Battalion of most Armies in the world. The Battalion should have a standardised list of medical equipment and specific packages for specific operations. In its aspiration to be a capable Medical Force, commanders must ensure that its logistics requirements are being met, maintained and enhanced.

12.2 Poor Communication Networks

Effective management of the Medical Battalion depends on the ability to communicate with the various chains of commands. The battalion must be provided with the latest state-of-the-art communication sets. All departments in the unit must be equipped with appropriate radio communication networks.

At the present scenarios, communication is a great problem. Some Armies have no integrated radio communication networks within the battalion and external communication with relevant Brigade and Divisional staff is limited.

> *"We need better inter-command networks to support our existence and enhance our readiness." (A8)*

> *"Even with good tactical and operational plan, we will not be able to function if there is an unreliable communication networks." (A1)*

> *"We often end up using our hand phones. Our ambulances have no radio-sets." (A2)*

> *"It is a 'hodgepodge' affair." (A1)*

In an operational environment, communication is essential to the success of the mission. Without communication there will be no coordination between units. Medical Support requests cannot be made, medical intelligence information cannot be transmitted and casualties cannot be evacuated.

Without communication, liaison with Medical Headquarters relating to staff replacement, logistics requirements, medical intelligence, supervision of operation, assignment of attached units, medical evacuation and referrals, blood management, medical resupply, medical maintenance, ground and air ambulance support will all fail. This situation is unimaginable if there is real war. In order to enhance communication, the Battalion must be provided with sufficient communication network facilities.

PART 6
Addressing the Readiness Factors

CHAPTER 13

OPERATIONAL AND TRAINING PERSPECTIVE

13.1 Develop Well Defined Operational Mission

Continuing to support OOTW will stress the battalion. At the moment, the Medical Battalion has been made to provide a whole spectrum of missions ranging from combat support to HADR operations and medical standby for sports. There is a need to develop standard criteria for deployment in order to clarify the missions and not to burden the unit.

Standard operating procedures and guidelines to cater for the different types of missions must be written and strictly followed. Rules of engagement for medical missions must be clarified. Commanders must abide to the deployment criteria and mission creeps must be avoided. There is a need to clarify upfront the mission objectives, concept of operations and types of patients eligible for treatment. Even if there are some political elements associated with OOTW, this can be handled tactfully by having a standardised deployment criteria approved by the highest authority.

13.2 Enhance Training

A new training department must be established by the battalion to cater for the training needs of the personnel. New curriculum must be developed to conduct regimental and medical courses tailored towards the training needs of the personnel. Training needs analysis must be done. New relevant courses related to Army Medicine such as Combat Trauma Life Support, Combat Casualty Care, Battlefield Medicine and other related courses must be developed and conducted. Training logs must be maintained.

Military doctors and medics must be trained to be able to:

a. be deployed anywhere, anytime and are able to serve in war and critical situations.
b. Understand the needs of the military profession and take part actively in health maintenance and well-being of the military community.
c. Handle patients in critical situations during war, disaster and mass casualty events.
d. Manage illness due to work hazards faced by military personnel such as special forces, drivers, paratroopers, pilots, etc.
e. Communicate and make decisions in challenging situations.

It is also worth considering the use of modeling and simulation to enhance medical readiness. Modeling and simulation enable medical commanders to set scenarios and conduct virtual training. This will enable medics to observe the various stage and processes that may happen in a real war. However, it will not give an actual impact of what is going to happen in real life. It will also not able to assess actual skills, morale, environment and tactics. It can be difficult, complex and time consuming.

It is important to develop new training methods and access to information must be made easily available. Training materials not affecting security must be reclassified and posted on the battalion website. This will enhance collaborative learning. Military style regimented training may not be applicable to medical skill training.

Adult learning approach need to be introduced. Combined learning modes, facilitated discussion, dialogue, simulation may all help to enhance learning. Special *train the trainer program* need to be conducted to enhance teaching and learning.

At the moment, training at the battalion is "ad-hoc". It mostly focuses on regimental training rather than enhancing medical skill. A balance must be made with the correct mix of regimental and clinical training programs. It is worth pursuing the establishment of the Centre for Disaster and Military Medicine proposed by the author in joint collaboration with Genesis and Canadian Aerospace (CAE). This Centre will incorporate latest technology in virtual reality. Medical simulation will be conducted under austere battlefield and disaster environments. Students practising the art of medicine will have visual, tactile, auditory and smell components incorporated in the training scenarios. They will have a chance to practise medicine under virtual jungle, desert, swamp, disaster, and other austere environment (see Figure 2, 3 and 4).

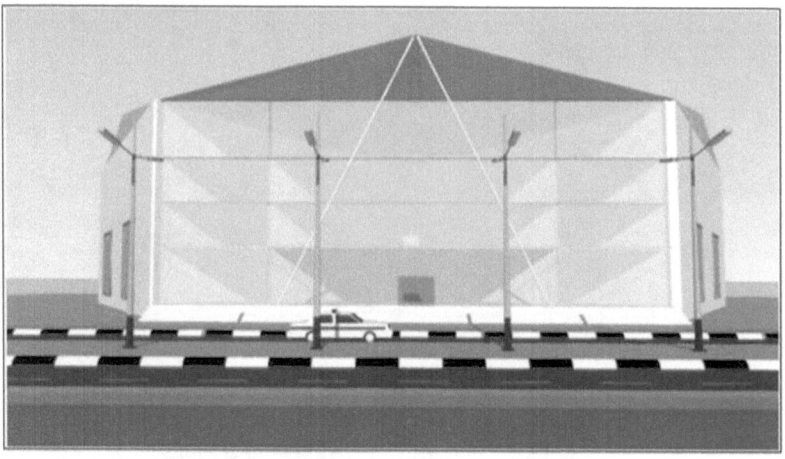

Figure 2: Disaster and Military Medicine Simulation Centre – Proposed Building

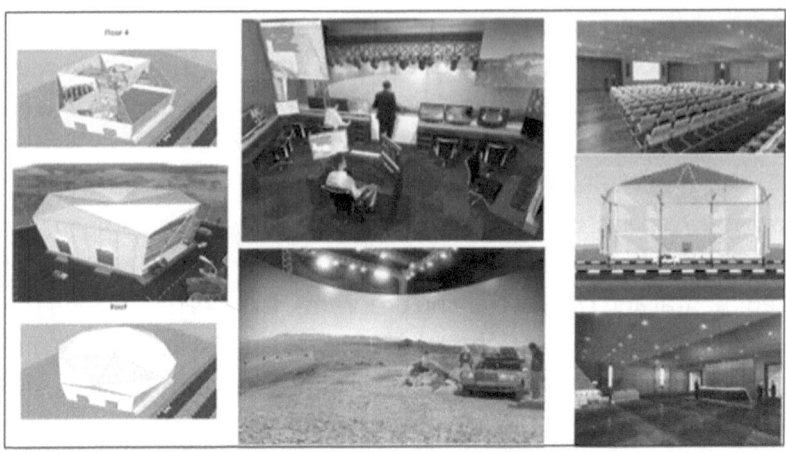

Figure 3: Training Facilities at the Disaster
and Military Medicine Simulation Centre

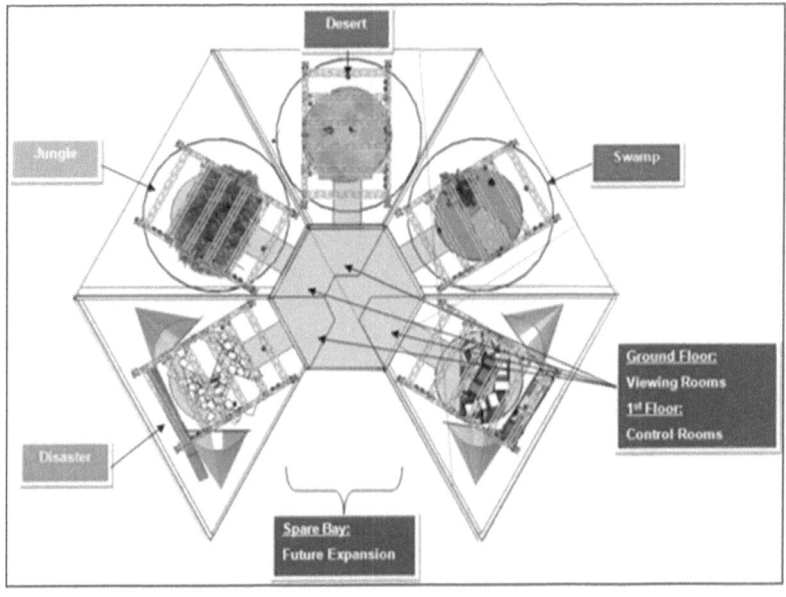

Figure 4: Floor Plan of the Disaster and Military
Medicine Simulation Centre Comprising Jungle,
Desert, Swamp and Disaster Environment

CHAPTER 14

ENHANCING MANAGEMENT

14.1 Change Management

In any organisation, more so in the military, getting top management commitment is an important requirement for changes to occur. It is important to create a sense of urgency on the subject of Medical Readiness as it affects National Security. The fact that the Medical Battalion is well known for its contributions in conflicts and disasters will make it more urgent for stakeholders to enhance Medical Readiness. Any shortfall on its capability will compromise the military's image.

Kotter's Change Management principles comprising eight steps approach in transforming organisation would be an appropriate strategy. There is a need here, as proposed by Kotter (2002) to:

a. Create sense of urgency on the critical situations and state of affairs of the battalion.
b. Build a guiding coalition among top, middle and low level management. Engage all key personnel in the Army to reduce barriers and form a network to enhance readiness.
c. Get the right vision: The vision and mission of the battalion must be re-examined taking into considerations the present political, environmental, social, legal, technological and environmental development (PESTLE).
d. Communicate the vision for buy-in: The new vision must be made known across all stakeholders, right from the

Minister of Defence and Chief of Army down to every officers and enlisted man of the division, brigade and battalion.

e. Empowers broad – based action: The Medical Battalion must be given greater authority to purchase, repair or maintain medical and non-medical equipment. The battalion commanding officer must be given more authority on matters concerning operations, administration and logistics.

f. Generate short term wins: Good performance must be recognised. Successful improvement processes and achievements in any forms must be made known to all. Contributions by the battalion in the various missions must be publicised. Recognitions should be given to all achievements made by individuals and groups. This will help to motivate staff and facilitate the change process.

g. Don't let up: Efforts to improve the state of affairs of the Medical Battalion have started since a long time ago, but most of them stalled due to lack of perseverance. Most improvement programmes stopped halfway. There was no continuity when leaders left, projects got stalled, and staff got demoralised. Battalion team members lack focus and perseverance in seeing projects through. Using the Balanced Scorecard approach with several K.P.I's will help steer the Battalion forward and ensure continuity of projects even if leaders leave.

h. Make it stick: New improvement processes must involve every members of the battalion. All change processes should be part of the Battalion's routine. Resilience among personnel must be cultured, stakeholders engaged and relationship enhanced. New work processes must be made known to everybody, and accomplishments rewarded where and when appropriate.

14.2 Balanced Scorecard

Another useful tool to get top management commitment is by developing a strategic plan dedicated to Army Medicine using the Balanced Scorecard method. This will help to align vision with operation and facilitate the change processes mentioned above. It helps to translate the organisation's vision and strategy into actions. The Medical Battalion aspires to be a world class provider of Military Health Care by delivering high quality services, developing and equipping a Medical Force with wartime operational capabilities, and training and developing medical personnel with regimental and wartime clinical skill (see Figure 5).

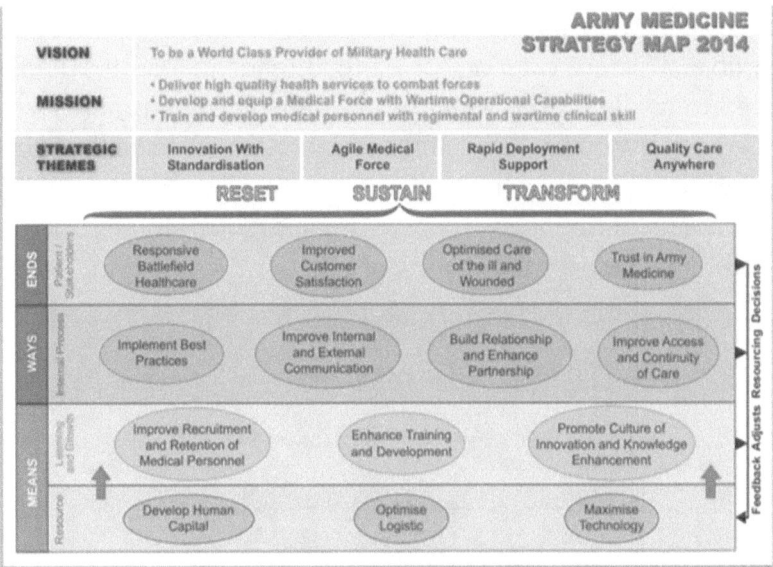

Figure 5: Army Medicine Strategy Map
(Adapted from various models)

14.3 Organisation Structure

The Medical Battalion must be restructured in accordance with the latest change in operational scenarios. Instead of the normal hierarchical organisation, there is a need to have a flatter organisation to cater for the different sub-specialties within the medical profession.

New medical departments within the Medical Battalion must be established to take into consideration current and future operational requirements. Future trends in military development, Revolutions in Military Affairs (RMA) and changes in medical technology will have profound effect on battlefield healthcare provision. Having different teams specialised for different operations will enhance the Battalion's readiness. A robust and flexible structure catering for a broad range of health services need to be designed to cater for the varied demands of military operations. Modular, highly mobile and self – contained medical units manned by emergency physicians should be incorporated in the new organisation. A proposed organisational structure of the Medical Battalion is shown in Figure 6.

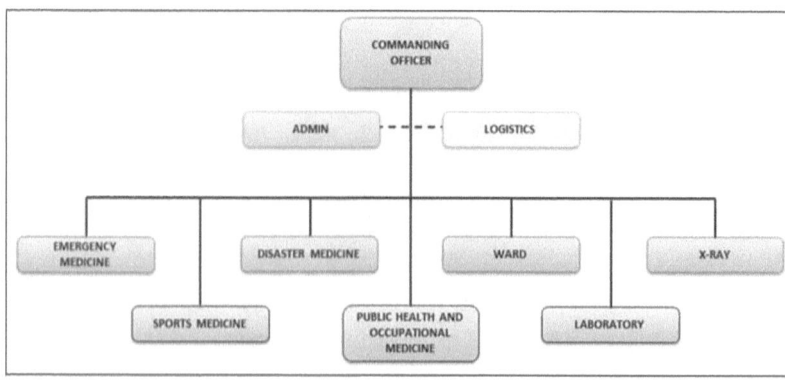

Figure 6: A Proposed Organisational Structure for a Medical Battalion

14.4 Improve Shortage of Personnel

The battalion requires the full complement of personnel with the correct types of specialty to properly function in demanding situations. Critical wartime personnel shortages must be addressed. Medical personnel must receive war-time combat related clinical skill training prior to deployment. Unit personnel readiness status must be regularly maintained and monitored. Availability of certain specialists must be ensured if particular deployments require certain expertise e.g. obstetrician, paediatricians, sports physicians etc. This is to cater for HADR missions and sports medical standby.

It is worth noting that shortages will severely affect readiness. Shortages in the critical specialties are perennial problems. One way to solve this is to engage the Medical Reserve Companies and mobilise them when required. Most countries have Medical Companies (Reserves) comprise several specialists who are eager to join the regular force for short term overseas missions. More Reserved Medical companies should be established at the civilian General Hospitals.

Shortages of Medical personnel will continue to exist and the figures could be greater. Many doctors and medics are on long study leave to obtain their specialist qualifications while some personnel are not deployable due to health reasons. Many others are not skilful while others are wrongly assigned for jobs they are not trained for. Good human resource management will go a long way in enhancing readiness.

CHAPTER 15

IMPROVING LOGISTIC AND COMMUNICATION

15.1 Enhance Logistic Support

The importance of logistics support cannot be over emphasized. Both army logistics and military healthcare supply chain must transform to cater for 21st century medical demand. Special purposed medical packages to cater for different needs of operations should be prepacked and deployed when needed. Technology and use of ICT must be enhanced. The Medical Corps, being a service support unit of the Army, must have a good concept of logistic support. This is to cater for ease of procurement, maintenance and repair of emergency equipment. Equipment must also be easily interchangeable so as to enhance interoperability between friendly nations. The military health care supply chain management projects proposed by Basari (2009), if adapted properly, can help to enhance supply chain in the Army. This comprehensive strategy consists of seven elements, namely partnership, training, negotiation, technology, standardisation, agility and deployment (see Figure 7).

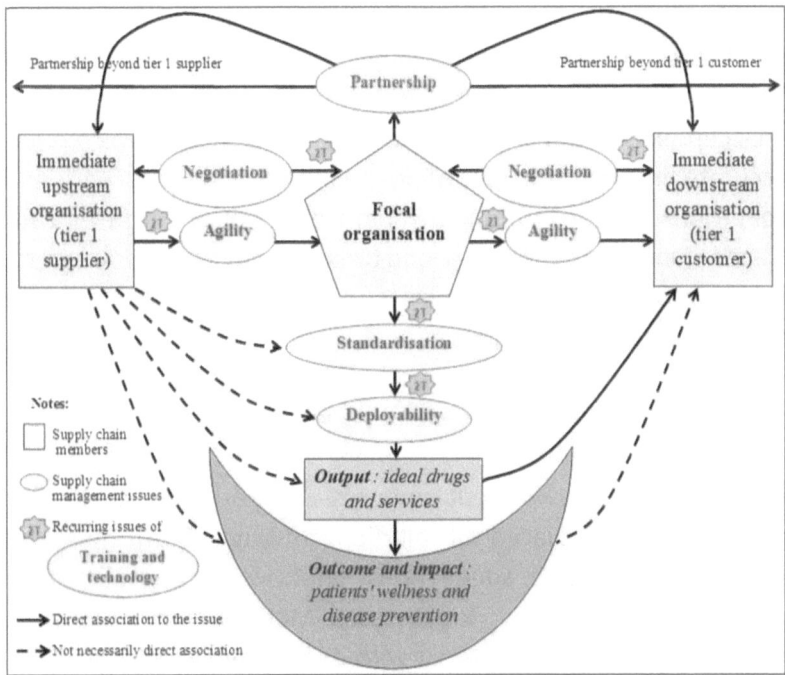

Figure 7: Seven Elements of Military Healthcare Supply Chain (Adopted from Basari, A.H.)

The Medical Corps being a service support unit must have a good concept of logistic support to cater for emergency requirements. Equipment must be easily interchangeable to enhance interoperability. Maintenance support plan must be continually updated.

15.2 Improve Communication Networks

Both military radio communication networks and interpersonal communication channels must be enhanced. Greater cooperation between stakeholders needs to be established. Rigid military systems that hinder communication must be removed.

More efforts should be made to equip the battalion with all the necessary communication equipment. Deployment of field ambulances without communication and navigation devices is unacceptable in the modern era. Rescue Medical Teams require accurate information regarding actual location and patient's conditions in order to render rapid treatment. Trying to locate places of incidents will take a long time without navigation assets. Furthermore, the *golden hours of injury management* requires casualties to be treated immediately.

Other than having good communication networks, commanders must also develop good communication skills. They must learn to be good listeners and facilitate exchange of information freely without unnecessary barriers. Suggestion boxes must be placed at all departments. Staff must be encouraged to give suggestions on how to improve work environment and the work processes. More opportunities must be created for staff to interact with each other. Meetings, when conducted, must be followed by feedback and recommendations must be implemented.

Communication will long continue to be a major challenge in military organisation. Improving military units' communication strategy will go a long way in moving the organisation forward.

PART 7
The Way Forward

CHAPTER 16

PLANNING FOR 21ST CENTURY MEDICAL READINESS

Planning is a complex process. It requires a rigorous multidisciplinary approach. Planning should be comprehensive, clear, practicable, future-oriented and consistent with the military commander's concept of operation. It must be configured to respond to the demands of present and future conflicts.

A good plan must be able to provide the necessary organisation and resources to accomplish the mission. It must be properly coordinated, flexible and provide for proper command and control. It must support the tactical commander's requirements. Sometimes it has to compromise between the number likely to be injured and the assets available.

Military health services must be able to function in an increasingly austere and dynamic environment. It should keep pace with the latest technological advances and cater for the increasing expectation of the stakeholders. Military health services must be robust, seamless and able to support the full spectrum of military operations. It must follow the principles of conformity, proximity, flexibility and mobility. A proper command and control structure must be established.

It is important for military health services to be well prepared, fully equipped, fully trained and ready to respond to any eventualities. Services provided must be of the highest quality, readily accessible, safe, sustainable and flexible enough to meet the changing needs of the operational environment. A high level of commitment by top management is critical to the success of the medical support operation.

In the 21st century, military healthcare is experiencing a rapid pace of innovations designed to improve quality, enhance access, eliminate waste, reduce harm and increase efficiency. Development of new technologies such as electronic health records, health wearables, telehealth, mobile technology, 3D printing and artificial intelligence can transform healthcare in the operational environment. Digital technology is changing the way healthcare is delivered and militaries worldwide should explore new methods to manage healthcare in the frontline. The future of healthcare is patient-centred, connected, mobile and precise. With soldiers at the top of our mind, we must look forward to harnessing the potential of technology as we resolve into this fascinating era of Industrial Revolution 4.0.

CHAPTER 17
CONCLUSION

This study focused on the readiness of a Medical Battalion as an Army unit in support of a Division. To begin with, PESTLE, SWOT and SOAR analysis were performed. A qualitative study was then conducted using the conceptual framework as shown earlier in Figure 1. Results were analysed and factors affecting medical readiness were identified. A Medical Readiness Concept Plan was developed as shown in Figure 8.

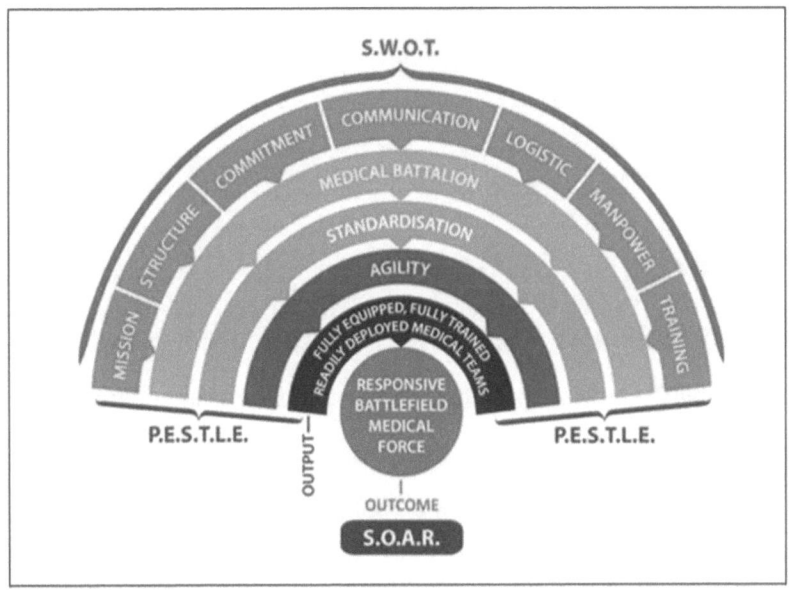

Figure 8: Medical Readiness Concept Plan

The study summarises factors affecting Medical Readiness which can be attributed to:

a. Inadequately defined mission.
b. Inadequate training.
c. Lack of top management commitment.
d. Out-dated organisational structure.
e. Shortage of manpower.
f. Poor logistics support.
g. Poor communication networks.

Recommendations to address the above factors are summarised in Table 2.

Ser	Problems	Recommendations
1	**G Factors**	
	a. Inadequately defined mission	Develop well defined operational mission
	b. Inadequate training	Enhance training
2	**A Factors**	
	a. Lack of top management commitment	Get top management commitment
	b. Out-dated organisational structure	Restructure the organisation
	c. Shortage of manpower	Improve shortage of personnel
3	**Q Factors**	
	a. Poor logistics support	Enhance logistic support
	b. Poor communication networks	Improve communication networks

Table 2: Medical Readiness Problems and Recommendations

It is important to develop a well-defined operational mission, enhance training, get top management commitment, restructure out-dated organisation, fill up shortages of personnel, enhance logistic support and improve communication networks. Addressing these seven factors will result in an agile, fully equipped, fully trained, and readily deployed medical team with a high state of readiness.

References

Air Force Instruction 10-250 (2007) Individual Medical Readiness, Department of Air Force, United States of America.

Australia. Department of DMS 3 MD Ex Golden Starlight Australia (1983) Medical Planning – Appreciation factor guide. Royal Australian Army Medical Corp, pp.1-5.

Basari, A. H. (2009) 'Military healthcare supply chain management: Malaysian armed forces perspectives', Under the Aegis of the International Committee Of Military Medicine 38 th World Congress on military medicine, Malaysia, 4-9 October.

Bellamy, R. F. and Llewellyn, C. H. (1990) Preventable Casualties: Rommel's Flaw, Slim's Edge, Army, 40 (5), pp. 52-56.

Bidin, M. Z. (1993) Health Services Support in Combat. Journal of The Malaysian Armed Forces Medical and Dental Corps, (1), pp. 4-7.

Grau, L. W. and Jorgensen, W. A. (1997) Beaten by the Bugs, the Soviet- Afghan war experience, Military Review 77(6), pp.30-37.

Jenkin, I. (2004) The Changing World of Military Healthcare, Journal of the Royal Army Medical Corps, (150), pp. 234-238.

Joseph, S. C. (1995) Maintaining cost effective military health care, U.S Department of Defense Office of the Assistant Secretary of Defense (Public Affairs). [Online]. Available from http://www.defense.gov/Speeches/Speech.aspx?SpeechID=969 [Accessed 17 November 2014].

Junor, L.J. (2005) The Defence Readiness Reporting System: A New Tool for Force Management, Joint Force Quarterly, 39.

Kasper, M. and Klein, L. (2000) Deployment Phase Medical Readiness Support Paper presented at the RTO HFM Specialist Meeting on The Impact of NATO International Military Missions on Health Care Management, held in Kiev, Ukraine, 4-6 Sept 2000 and published in RTO MP-068.

Lloyd, J. (undated) Organizational structure can be underlying causes of workplace issues. [Online]. Available from: http://www.jobdig.com/articles/439/Organizational_structure_can_be_underlying_cause_of_workplace_issues.html [Available from 11 November 2014].

Nor, N. A. M. (2003) Measurement of capability and readiness of Army Unit, Department of Army, Kuala Lumpur, Malaysian Army Journal.

Peltz, E. et al (2002) Diagnosing the Army's Equipment Readiness- The Equipment Downtime Analyzer, RAND Arroyo Center, Santa Monica, pp.1-82.

Picturesque Expressions: A Thematic Dictionary, 1(1980) 1st ed. The Gale Group, Inc.

Random House Kernerman Webster's College Dictionary (2010) K Dictionaries Ltd, Random House.

Salisbury, D. and English, A. (2003) Prognosis 2020: Military Medical Strategy for the Canadian Forces, Canadian Military Journal, 4 (2), pp.45-54.

The American Heritage Dictionary of the English Language. (2000) 4th ed. Houghton Mifflin Company.

United Kingdom. Royal Army Medical Corps, RAMC History. [Online]. Available from: http://www.ams-museum.org.uk/museum/history/ramchistory/ [Accessed 16 November 2014].

United States General Accounting Office Report to Congressional Requesters, (1995) Defense Health Care – Issues and Challenges Confronting Military Medicine, GAO/HEHS-95-104, pp. 1-34.

United States of America. (2012) Department of The Army, Navy Air Force, Health Service Support, Joint Publication 4-02, pp.13-16

INDEX

A

Administrative (A) factor, 37, 38, 39, 74
Agility, 66
Armed Forces Hospital, 10
Army Medical Corps, 16
Army Medicine, 58, 63

B

Balanced Scorecard, 62, 63
Battlefield Environment, 3
Battlefield Medicine, 58

C

Canadian Aerospace, 59
Casualties, 8
Casualty Estimate, 18
Center for Disaster and Military Medicine, 59
Change Management, 61, 62
Climate, 17
Combat Casualty Care, 58
Combat Medical Service, 3
Combat Multiplier, 3
Combat Trauma Life Support, 58
Communication Networks, 40, 53, 54, 67, 68, 74
Conformity, 10
Continuity, 10
Control, 10

D

Defence Medical Outputs, 7
Disaster and Military Medicine Simulation Centre, 59, 60

E

Echelons of Care, 9, 10
EME, 47, 50
Enemy Situation, 17

F

Field Ambulance, 68
Field Hospital, 9
Field Surgical and Transfusion Team, 47
First Responder, 9
Flexibility, 10
Flora and Fauna, 17
Forward Resuscitative Care, 9
Friendly Situation, 17

G

General Rommel, 7
Genesis, 59
Golden Hours, 68

H

HADR, 57
Health of Troops, 18
Hepatitis, 7

I

Interoperability, 66

L

Logistic, 50, 51, 52, 53, 66, 71, 74
Logistic (Q) factor, 37, 38, 39, 40, 74

M

Management Commitment, 45, 74
Management Initiatives, 20, 71
Manpower, 48, 49
Medical Battalion, 9, 15, 25, 26, 27, 30, 31, 45, 46, 47, 48, 49, 50, 53, 62, 63, 64
Medical Planning Checklist, 16, 17, 18, 19
Medical Readiness
    Components, 32
    Conceptual Framework, 37, 38, 39, 40
    Factors, 22, 30, 31, 45, 46
    Individual, 29, 31
    Meaning, 25, 29, 30, 31
    Measure, 26, 27
Medical Corps, 66
Medical Packages, 66
Military Doctors, 45, 58
Military Healthcare, 20, 21, 22, 63, 71, 72
Military Healthcare Supply Chain, 66, 67
Mission, 41, 74
Mobility, 10
Mobilization Plan, 71
Modelling and Simulation, 58
Morale, 3

N

Nature of Operation, 16

O

OOTW, 57
Operational (G) factor, 37, 38, 39, 74
Operational Mission, 57
Operational Plan, 32
Ordnance, 47
Organisation Structure, 47, 48, 64, 74

P

Personnel, 49, 65, 74
PESTLE, 21, 61, 72, 73
Preventive Medical Measures, 32, 33
Principles of Health Services Support, 9
Proximity, 10

R

Rapid Development Force, 7
Readiness, 8, 61, 74, 71, 72
Regimental Aid Post, 15
Regimental Medical Officer, 7, 9
Reserved Medical Companies, 65
Resources, 18
Revolution in Military Affairs, 64

S

Service Corps, 47
SOAR, 72, 73
Soviet Afghan War, 7
Standardisation, 66, 73
Strength to be Supported, 17

SWOT, 72, 73

T

Technology, 66
Terrain, 17
Time and Space, 18
Training, 42, 43, 66

U

USA Department of Army, 10, 16, 52
US General Accounting Office, 20, 22, 71

www.ingramcontent.com/pod-product-compliance
Lightning Source LLC
Chambersburg PA
CBHW022116170526
45157CB00004B/1669